I0792016

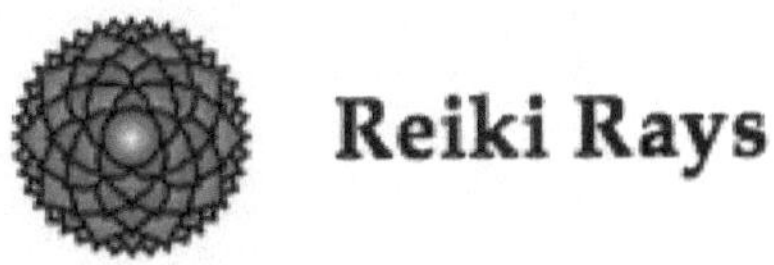

When Spirit Meets Science

Empowered Healing for the New Age

Haripriya Suraj
& Suraj Manjunath

Copyright

© 2020, Acorn Gecko SRL

ALL RIGHTS RESERVED. This book contains material protected under International and Federal Copyright Laws and Treaties. Any unauthorized reprint or use of this material is prohibited. No part of this book may be reproduced or transmitted in any form or by any means, electronic or mechanical, including photocopying, recording, or by any information storage and retrieval system without express written permission from the publisher.

Table of Contents

Preface

This work is an outcome of a decade long intense interaction between two different personalities – one rational and one intuitive. We view every relationship as a teacher. And this book is the result of what our relationship taught us, along our journey as soul partners.

When we set foot on our personal journey together, we had no clue that our starkly contrasting approaches to reality would lead to the birth of a new idea and serve as a stepping stone into a new age. We believe that this idea, which is a marriage of science and spirituality, holds great promise for humanity.

The path was certainly not an easy one to walk on, for it was filled with angst, turmoil, shocks, surprises and never ending debates. But in hindsight, it seems well worth the deeper learning and growth that unfolded along the way. The tumultuous journey carved itself into a middle path that embraces the best of Spirit and Science. It transformed the question of *'Spirit or Science?'* to the answer *'Spirit and Science.'*

To us, the biggest reward presented by the journey was the discovery of unconditional love - the joy of loving a person for who they are and honoring their purpose for what it is.

This book provides the best of intuitive insights and scientific knowledge to anyone who would like to explore a combined approach to healing. It is an exploration of both sides of the coin.

The first part of the book describes our personal story of the discovery of Spirit through Reiki and Science through Medicine. It also shares the insights we received as we each traversed our individual and collective paths.

The second part of the book shares information on research methodology. It gives a glimpse into the world of research and serves as a useful foundation for those practitioners of alternative therapies who would like to engage in high quality scientific research.

The third part of the book is more metaphysical in nature. It shares a vision for a new model of healing and medicine. This model is based on the best of intuitive wisdom and scientific inquiry. It offers a peek into a dream that we hope will manifest as reality on Planet Earth.

We are grateful to everyone who has been part of our journey - our families, our spiritual and academic teachers, the wider community of energy healers and medical doctors who have all played a role in the creation of this work, and to the mighty forces of Spirit and Science.

We are grateful to Maria Diaconu for her unconditional support and to the entire Reiki Rays team for helping this book reach the world.

And our heartfelt gratitude to you, Dear Reader! We feel honored to be sharing this book with you. We trust you will receive everything you need from this work to enrich and support your own journey.

Haripriya and Suraj

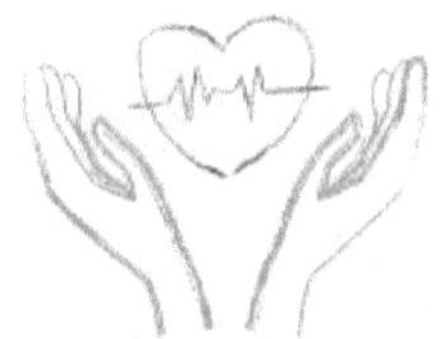

Part 1

Intuitive Ms. Feminine

and

Rational Mr. Masculine

The Seed of Reiki
Haripriya

Oh, beautiful Reiki,

Of rainbow colors bright.

What a wonder you are,

Though nowhere in sight!

They say a child's world is filled with wonder and magic!

Children are more open to experiencing miracles that lie outside the realm of third dimensional reality.

I got a peek into the world of Reiki when I was a child. And for this I am very grateful. I believe this childhood peek helped me view this beautiful energy with a sense of pure wonder and delight.

It was during my visits to a close friend's home that I was introduced to Reiki. I often saw my friend's mother standing near her plants, with her palms over them, keenly focused. When I asked my friend what was going on, she told me that her mother was giving energy to the plants and that it was called Reiki.

I was intrigued by what I witnessed those days. It was like the first seed of Reiki was sown within me, probably a deeper knowing stirred on a very subconscious level.

The Reiki Connection

Many souls in the healing community feel a connection with Reiki, that seems to go beyond space, time and logic. Maybe it's the word Reiki that strikes a chord. Or the idea of connecting with an energy that is expansive and universal; an energy that we hope will bring peace to a racing mind, love to a broken heart or purpose to a lost soul. Some souls inclined to esoteric wisdom also trace this connection to past lifetimes in which they may have incarnated as healers.

No matter how Reiki comes into one's life, it is a sacred connection and a very special beginning.

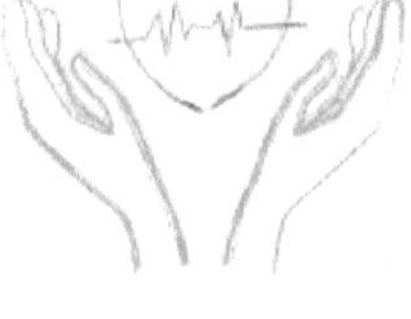

The Seed of Science
Suraj

Science is God,

God is Science.

Hail the logical mind,

A gift to humankind.

Rational thinking and logic have been an intrinsic part of my life for as long as I can remember. It was something that I accepted as the norm, not just for me but for most of the world.

Being a student of science helped me explore the world of logic on a deeper level. Medical training took it several notches higher. Diagnosis and treatment protocols that we offered to patients were the result of logical, unbiased scientific research performed in highly systematic ways.

Training in research methodology expanded the horizons of my mind. I discovered a new love and passion for scientific research. And I learnt to apply logic and scientific thinking to many aspects of my life, not just to medical practice.

The Gifts of Science

People living in the 21st century are privileged to experience the marvels of science. From the electricity that lights up homes to the vaccinations that have eradicated deadly diseases, from air travel to the mobile phone, every discovery and invention have been the result of thorough scientific exploration of brilliant ideas.

Observation, experimentation and deduction are the hallmarks of the scientific method. Every idea is subjected to rigorous testing and verification before it is finally presented as fact to the world. When you sit in an airplane, you know for certain that it can do its job of transporting you to your destination. When one is given a local anesthetic for tooth extraction, the removal of the tooth is expected to be almost painless.

Thanks to high quality research, there is no second guessing as to the result delivered by scientific discoveries and inventions.

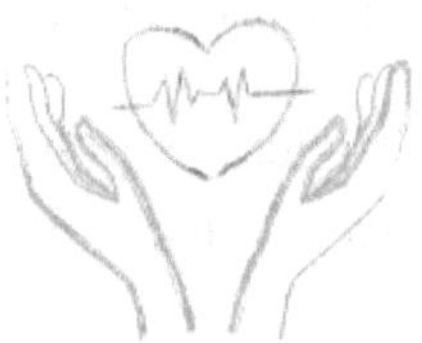

When Reiki comes Knocking at the Door
Haripriya

Little seed, full of might

Sprout you must when the time is right!

I faced numerous challenges as I transitioned from childhood to teenage to adulthood, with relationships taking the hardest beating of all. I was on a roller coaster, being tossed from challenge to challenge. In my early twenties, I was in the midst of one such challenge, battling fears and phobias on the one hand and a relationship breakdown on the other hand. This is when a deep desire to learn Reiki surfaced in me.

As the saying goes, *"When the student is ready, the teacher appears."*

And I was led to my Reiki teacher in perfect time. When I set foot into her abode, harboring a strong intention to connect with Reiki, I felt like a part of me was home. Things unfolded quickly and I moved from receiving a healing session to receiving my first attunement within a month's time.

Connecting with Reiki brought me immense peace, joy, and bliss. It was an experience unlike anything I had ever had in my life. As a newly attuned Reiki channel, I was extremely sensitive to the energy flowing through my being. I thoroughly enjoyed the sensations of my palms heating up, when placed over certain areas of the body.

My teacher told me that Reiki has a way of clearing out clutter (unhelpful patterns, relationships, things and situations) from our lives. Truly enough, in the midst of the 21-day self-healing process (a three-week period of daily self-Reiki that practitioners strictly adhere to after getting attuned to a level of Reiki), the relationship challenge I was facing began to dissipate. The relationship received closure, bringing much needed healing, in the form of lessons learnt and wisdom gained.

The Blessing of Reiki

In Japanese, 'Rei' means universal and 'Ki' means life force energy. Energy healers understand that Reiki is the divine life force which animates the physical body and keeps the chakras and energy field in balance. It is a relaxing and balancing energy that promotes wellness and harmony.

When we go deeper into Reiki practice, some of us discover that it also works towards clearing our lives of anything that does not serve our greater good.

How does Reiki do this? And what has this got to do with health, wellness and balance?

The answer stems from the higher understanding that we are much more than our physical bodies. Health is not restricted to our physical body alone but encompasses our mental, emotional and spiritual aspects as well.

Therefore, Reiki is automatically connected to every aspect of our existence and works to bring about overall balance. Just as the body's immune system works to eliminate germs, Reiki works to remove blocks and obstacles, so that we align with our highest potential.

Reiki is a beautiful blessing in our lives!

Medicine Calling
Suraj

Call it free will or fate,

Set up with medicine on a lifelong date.

A new way of life to live,

Where it's all about give, give and give.

Give treatment, give time, give hope,

Even when tired and at the end of the rope.

Groomed and polished, by night and day,

Until a fine doctor become one may.

I did not enter the medical profession by choice or because it was a passion. Medicine was merely a promising career option available when I was seventeen. The results of aptitude tests that I wrote opened up doors for my entry into medical school. Neither happy nor sad, I accepted my new role and decided to make the most of it.

Once into the course, the reality of the training dawned on me. It was hard work and certainly not for the faint at heart. It demanded rigorous study at the under-grad levels. It was even more demanding at the post grad and higher levels. In between taking care of patients and studying, there was hardly any time to rest or eat a meal in peace.

Considering that India was relatively less developed in the nineties, medical training often required working in less than optimal healthcare settings and treating an overwhelmingly large number of patients each day. This led to fatigue and burnout, not to mention compromise on time spent with family, friends, hobbies and passions. I kept at it despite all the challenges faced along the way and worked hard throughout. To my logical mind, once in medicine, I had better do the best I could, and accept things that couldn't be changed.

At the end of a training period spanning a long fourteen years, I was all set to be an independent consultant in surgical oncology.

Medicine: A Combination of Science and Art

• Medical training enables one to gain firsthand experience of the scientific method. From dissection of the human body in the first year to delivery of babies in the final year, plenty is available for a student to see, experience and learn hands on.

• The treatments offered are largely evidence based and scientifically proven

• The benefits as well as side effects of every medicine/ procedure are well documented. There is no sugar coating.

• The skill of a clinician lies in making a reasonably accurate diagnosis and offering a suitable treatment plan for an individual patient.

• A treatment is offered only when its benefits to the patient far outweigh the risks that it poses – and this often requires clinical judgement.

• Medicine is a combination of science and art. Diseases are as complex as the human body and their diagnosis and treatment can be quite challenging. Every treatment is offered in context, after evaluating the benefits and risks.

The Magic of New Beginnings
Haripriya

As the old falls apart,

The new touches the heart.

Magic and mystery abound.....

Prince of Masculine, he's found.

As the old made its way out of my life, I could sense the magic of new beginnings in the air!

Around the time that I completed my 21 day self-healing process, divine synchronicity waved its wand and my partner Suraj magically appeared in my life.

The first time I looked into his eyes, I felt a deep recognition. My logical mind couldn't explain it, but my soul understood it. He was every bit the partner I was working to manifest in my life. We were a great vibrational match, sharing similar values, likes and preferences. Very soon, we realized we were meant to be together and in a few months' time, we were man and wife!

The more I connected with Suraj, the more amazed I was at the way the Universe had brought him into my life. It was the first time in my life that I grew conscious of my ability to manifest something. Reiki prepared me energetically for this conscious manifestation.

Life Transitions and Conscious Manifestation

Endings and beginnings are a part of everyone's life. Working on ourselves energetically makes us more conscious of every ending and beginning we may encounter in life. It also helps us navigate these shifts with greater awareness and understanding.

Every ending offers lessons and wisdom, while every beginning brings with it new potential and possibilities. When we are aware, we assimilate the wisdom from the old and embrace the joy of the new. Rather than being tossed around by circumstances, we take responsibility and co-create our lives in alignment with our higher self. Conscious manifestation is a choice that is presented to us as we progress on this spiritual journey.

The Logic of New Beginnings
Suraj

The old precedes the new,

As does sunshine after the dew.

An order so natural,

Across all of life eternal.

As my professional life soared, my personal life was rooted in relationship challenges. After the meltdown of dysfunctional relationships, I was content to be all on my own for some time. I chose to allow life to take its own course until one fine day, I met my partner Haripriya.

I took an instant liking to her. My first conversation with her felt like a whiff of refreshing air that had come my way after eons. We built a great rapport in a very short time and took the happy decision to spend our lives together.

While we seemed to be alike in most respects, I found it intriguing that Haripriya spoke of energy and vibration in the context of everyday life. I only knew what these terms meant in the context of science and it took me a while to understand what Haripriya meant by these words. Her email address at the time was <u>positivevibesonly@...com.</u> And I must admit I was baffled when I first received an email from her rather unusual email address!

When Haripriya spoke about the magic that had brought us together, I honestly had no clue what she was talking about. I was happy to see her excitement about this 'magic' in her life. But from my end, her appearance in my life was something which just happened because of a combination of effort and chance. All I knew was that I liked her and was happy to spend my life with her.

Logic in Life and Love

Life presents numerous choices in every moment. Doors close from time to time and new doors open. There is always more than one option to choose from, and more than one path to explore. The chosen path depends upon what makes the most logical sense at that point in time.

Once a path has been chosen, it is all about enjoying the scenery that is present along the way. If mountains are found when one expected to find an ocean, wisdom lies in climbing the mountain anyway. And joy lies in enjoying the climb! You never know what treasures may be found up there. There is great freedom in the acceptance of life and everything it brings one's way.

Being logical works well for many.

And ever so often, the best logical decision is also the most intuitive one.

A Peek into the World of Physical Science and Rationality

Haripriya

Logic, logic,

Show thy magic!

Science divine

What a blessing art thine,

Divinity, oh love

Thee a mighty spirited dove,

Oh great Science and Sprit,

Why must thou part adrift?

During the initial days of our courtship, I understood Suraj to be a scientific and rational person. I attributed this to the fact that he was a highly qualified cancer surgeon, trained in evidence based medicine and experienced in advanced scientific research. Though I was deeply lodged in the world of subtle energy and intuition, I was perfectly comfortable with his scientific temperament.

However, I did have a subtle ego, which made me view his path as one which was inferior to mine. I assumed that people who were purely scientific and rational were narrow minded and closed to the mysteries of the Universe. I also believed that they were missing out on so much fun and goodness as their world was limited to the experience of the five senses.

My friends in the Reiki community told me that it wouldn't be long before the rational folks of the scientific community realize that their approach doesn't create lasting effects. Their words further stoked my ego. I was certain that my partner would yield one day and I would have the last word!

I waited and waited until one day I was forced to listen to the non-egoic murmurs of my heart and embrace a wider perspective......

The Tug of War between Science and Spirit

With the rapid advancement of science, there seems to have developed a tug of war between the worlds of science and spirit. Thousands of people world over, spend enormous amounts of time and effort debating the two disciplines.

Many in the energy and alternative healing community are critical of science, and modern medicine in particular. Modern medicine and the pharmaceutical industry are viewed with suspicion. Conventional medical treatments are often labelled as toxic and treating only the symptoms, while doing nothing to cure the root cause of illness.

On the other hand, many in the scientific and medical community are skeptical of anything that lies outside the realm of science and disparaging of the people who practice it. Alternative and energy therapies are dismissed as mumbo jumbo, lunacy, placebo, sham or sheer figment of imagination.

What would happen if people from both communities could put the ego aside and look at things with an open mind and heart? Not accept the other's view blindly, but at least be open to the possibility that each path may offer something good.

What if the world opened up to the possibility of Spirit and Science bringing the best of both their worlds together?

It would be the merging of the 'Rational Masculine' with the 'Intuitive Feminine.'

Imagine the beauty that would envelop such a world!

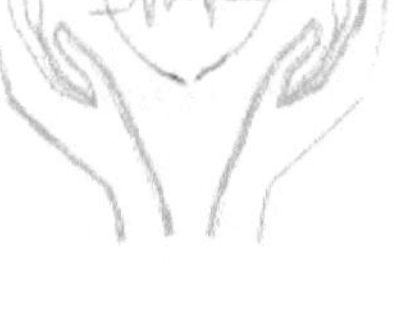

A Peek into the World of Spirit
Suraj

Spirit as God, the unknown,

Was the only version known.

A mighty force or a white bearded being?

Cannot say for sure without seeing.

Spirit as life force energy,

A new aspect of the universal synergy?

Logic bells refuse to ring,

Reiki nevertheless unfolds its wings.

During our courtship days, I came in contact with a few of Haripriya's friends practicing Reiki. As I interacted with them, I was shown a perspective that was diametrically opposite to my concept of reality. Her friends would talk of some unique applications of Reiki, such as clearing traffic jams, charging electronic devices, inducing weather changes and the like, all achieved through the assistance of Reiki! I was surprised and amused at the same time; surprised because I had never heard of such phenomena and amused to witness the casual way they were discussed, as though they were the commonest thing in the world!

The fact that Haripriya was a Reiki practitioner, was well received by my family. My grandmother knew about Reiki and had also got a taste of it earlier in life. She was excited to know that Haripriya could perform Reiki and she promptly set up weekly sessions with her. She eagerly looked forward to these Reiki sessions and couldn't stop talking about how relaxed and wonderful she felt after every session.

Over time, I understood Reiki to be a gentle and safe therapy that promotes relaxation and brings on feelings of wellness. I could not comprehend the mechanism behind it or find solid evidence to attest to its validity but the soothing effects of a Reiki healing on people were obvious enough to be seen.

If people found joy and spiritual connection through Reiki, I was happy for them!

Quest for Spirit

• Spirit is about finding the well of strength within oneself. As the quote goes- "Happiness is an inside job."

• Spirit is found in a beautiful sunrise and in the millions of stars adorning the night sky.

• Spirit is found in the majestic gait of the tiger and the graceful movements of the peacock.

• Spirit is found in the blankness of the mind, in the zone of nothingness.

• Spirit is found in the company and love of family and friends.

• Spirit is found in a beautiful work of art or a melodious piece of music.

• Spirit is found in the innocence of a young child.

• Spirit is found in the richness of new experiences.

• Spirit is found in non-judgement and acceptance of all humanity.

• Spirit is found in the art of doing nothing or simply being.

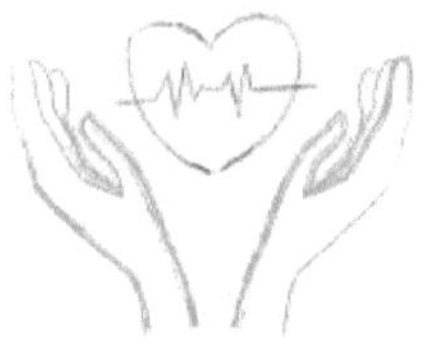

Conflicting Stories lead to Inner Dilemmas
Haripriya

Reiki flowing through the body's blocks,

Can it shatter tumors as hard as rocks?

Science asking for evidence if any,

Dismissing stories of miracles oh so many.

Hoping and aspiring high,

Then dropping low with a despondent sigh,

In the frenzy to eagerly show,

That which we may not fully know.

Hurting deep down inside,

Running from Reiki, seeking to hide,

Letting go with a broken heart,

Allowing the unknown to simply depart.

As a level 1 Reiki practitioner, I viewed Reiki as a magic pill that had solutions to all problems on Earth.

In the local Reiki community here, we often heard stories of people who were supposedly cured of illnesses such as cancer, hypertension and diabetes through Reiki alone. I was excited to share these stories with Suraj, in the hope that he would be thrilled to hear about these miraculous healings. But I was shocked and upset when each of these stories was lovingly yet firmly dismissed by my beloved partner. Nothing I said could impress or convince him.

To make matters worse, for every story of a miracle Reiki cure, he presented a perfectly valid scientific case as to why it couldn't be as claimed. Or he would ask to meet the person who was supposedly cured along with all medical reports as evidence. And this never materialized because most of the stories were verbal reports of what happened to people we didn't know or could never meet. In the few instances that reports were available, they did not correlate with the claims being made.

As time went by, I began to feel powerless. I had nothing to support my stance while Suraj had dozens of his own patients who suffered miserably for having denied conventional medical treatment in favor of other supposedly 'gentler therapies'.

Though the ego aspect of me wanted to disprove Suraj and his scientific logic, a part of me tuned into some truth behind his words.

During this time, I also received my Reiki level two attunement. The attunement was followed by a major healing crisis. I was revisited by old fears and phobias and they came in at a much higher intensity than ever before. Though I was guided to go within and stay with the process, I did not have the wisdom yet to do so. It felt extremely challenging and I just wanted the fears to go away and leave me alone. I was hoping my daily Reiki practice would make them go away. But they persisted. I then turned to pranic healing for additional support. But that didn't make them go away either.

My insistence that my fears MUST go away and my lack of preparation to look deeper into them created a huge block to healing. This, coupled with all that was happening to misguided patients at Suraj's hospital, drove me into the depths of despair. I was convinced that something was terribly wrong and that Reiki was probably not for me after all. I did not wish to be associated with therapies that could neither cure my mental fears nor the physical afflictions of the patients consulting my partner.

And one fine day, in the summer of 2008….

Reiki just disappeared from my life.

I let it go.

I let it go for I could not understand it.

I let it go for I could not prove it.

I let it go for it seemed like a huge battle to fight in the face of solid evidence based medicine.

I let it go because it began to feel like a burden to carry.

I let it go with a feeling of being let down.

I let it go with a heavy heart.

And out it went….

Reiki Disappearances

Reiki has a way of disappearing from peoples' lives.

One of the commonest reasons people give for their disconnect from Reiki is that their expectations were not fulfilled by it. Many of us embark on the Reiki path, in the hope that it will clean out every area of our lives; dissolve our mental and emotional issues, transform relationship troubles, cure physical health problems and make dreams come true.

And guess what happens when things don't happen as expected? Disappointment looms large and out goes Reiki through the window!

What if we have no predefined expectations of Reiki?

What if we explore it instead with a sense of curiosity and awe?

What if we allow Reiki to reveal itself to us?

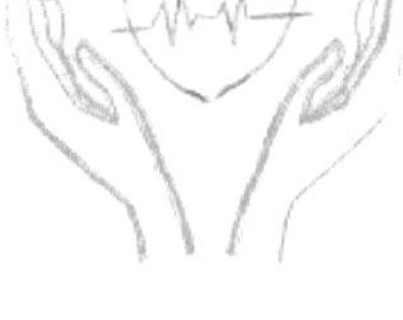

Conflicting Stories lead to Inner Turmoil
Suraj

Stories of miracles in the air,

Seek to comprehend what is rare.

Evidence to be found though none,

Alas, the damage is already done.

Going to a great many lengths,

To show good evidence is a sign of strength.

A service to provide confidence immense,

To the bodies in sickness oh so tense.

As I contemplated the unique perspectives and stories of my new friends in the energy healing community, I marveled at the fact that it takes all kinds to make the world. I was happy to embrace everyone without judgement, until one day, stories of Reiki medical miracles began to do the rounds. To me, this was a huge red flag.

Being a surgeon who works with cancer patients day in and day out, I had seen many cases of people opting for 'miracle cures.' Many would come back after some days, with worsening of the disease, sometimes from a curable to an incurable stage. As far as medical treatment for cancer goes, the earlier it is delivered the better. And it makes it challenging when people choose to delay treatment till the disease is advanced.

With all of this happening, it simply did not feel right when practitioners spoke casually about their personal Reiki treatments having cured people of serious medical conditions such as cancer and diabetes and epilepsy. There seemed to be no convincing evidence for any of this. And if some evidence was produced, there were plenty of holes in the claims which could not be plugged.

There was no doubt about the noble intentions of these practitioners. All of them were genuinely eager to help those who reached out to them in suffering. But was the healing they were offering truly helping patients overcome cancer or other major illnesses? And did these practitioners have any idea of the repercussions when it failed to heal as they believed it to?

Medical Miracles: Fact or Fiction

One of the most common accusations levelled by practitioners of other healing modalities against modern medicine is that it eradicates the symptoms of an illness, while doing nothing to heal a disease at the root. It is viewed as invasive, aggressive in its approach, not to mention toxic.

On the contrary, any form of supposedly 'natural healing' is viewed as safe, non-toxic and gentle on the body. And this is the very reason a lot of people turn to gentler therapies for healing support.

Natural is good of course. For instance, natural is great when it comes to eating seasonal fruits and vegetables, breathing in fresh air, not depending on unnecessary medication and allowing the body to heal itself naturally whenever it can. But natural may not be the best solution every time.

Each individual has the right to choose a treatment modality for himself. And if it works for him, well and good.

But what happens when it does not work?

It is disheartening when people who dismiss conventional treatment return to it in fear when other therapies do not work for them as hoped for.

Modern medicine may not seem natural in its approach and may not be able to cure every illness. But it certainly does an amazing job as far as management of many illnesses is concerned. A person with hypertension or diabetes may not be "cured" of the condition. But in most cases, it is possible for the condition to be managed effectively so the patient has a great chance of a near normal life.

As for toxicity, the benefits and side effects of every treatment are rigorously documented. There is always an element of risk in every treatment, just as for everything else in life. But considering the bigger picture, the benefits offered are almost always greater than the risks.

It has to be accepted that some treatments are invasive. After all, no one likes to be poked and prodded, cut open or experience physical discomfort. But the fact remains that all of this is done for a purpose and not with the intention of harming a patient. The benefits of surgical removal of a ruptured appendix far outweigh the damage it can cause if left untreated. A caesarean section is certainly not a natural way to give birth. But in cases where the life of the baby or the mother is endangered, the benefits of the procedure far outweigh the risks of allowing labor to progress naturally. An antihypertensive drug may carry a host of side effects but the benefits it offers outweigh the possible risks of cardiac illness/stroke if left untreated.

Medical miracles are welcome by all means! But before accepting a miracle as a given and charging forth to receive it, it may help to verify if there is substantial evidence to support a claim, especially when human lives are at stake.

For those in the giver's position, creating a solid evidence base before offering any form of therapy as medical treatment, will lend greater credibility to it. A research based approach will help to clarify if a particular healing modality helps in a specific illness and if yes, the ways in which it helps. This is something that every healing modality owes to those who look up to it with hope and trust.

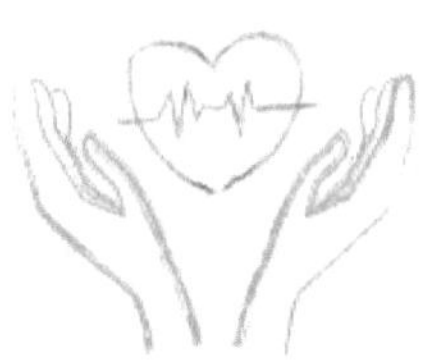

Is it Reiki vs Modern Medicine?
Haripriya

A few questions for healers to ponder-

• What are my core objectives when I offer energy healing to someone in physical, mental, emotional or spiritual pain?

• Since the energy body and the physical body are connected, can energetic health and physical health coexist yet receive different treatments if required?

• Am I authorized to make a medical diagnosis or to offer medical advice for the treatment of the physical body?

• Am I unconsciously in competition with modern medicine? Do I despise it on an unconscious level?

• If I carry negative beliefs around conventional healthcare, what would happen if I transform them into something higher?

• Can I allow myself to acknowledge the positive aspects of conventional healthcare? What kind of energy would this lend to healthcare?

• Can I view the benefits and risks that form a part of conventional healthcare from a higher and larger perspective?

• What would happen if a whole new integrative model of health and healing emerges, with different systems of healing contributing their unique strengths? Can I allow myself to dream of this possibility?

   • Can elements of research and structure be brought into intuitive forms of healing? Can elements of softness and compassion be brought into conventional healthcare?

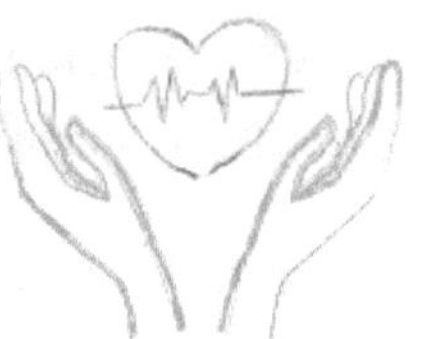

Modern Medicine to the Rescue
Haripriya

Science and research joining hands,

To offer healing across lands.

Pills and potions, syringes and knives,

Lend another chance to a zillion lives.

Harsh and stony as it may sound,

Evokes gratitude when other cures aren't found.

Soon after I let Reiki go, my life took on a very different flavor. I was deeply involved in day to day ground reality. I worked as a teacher in school, took care of a home that I grew to cherish and explored the world of love and marriage.

I then went on to conceive a beautiful child. Unexpectedly, towards the latter part of the pregnancy, my body manifested a major complication that stalled the growth of the baby. The condition turned into a medical emergency and we were left with no choice but to let our little baby girl go.

The letting go was agonizing in every sense of the word; firstly, the physical pain of labor only to deliver a child that I knew would come out lifeless, secondly, the mental agony of going through this experience in a cold and unfriendly hospital environment, thirdly, the emotions of loss and grief and lastly, the spiritual anguish of why I had manifested this experience despite being in the pink of health.

Even in the midst of my trauma, I found myself feeling grateful for the timely medical care that saved my life. The condition, if left untreated, could have endangered my own life. This is the time when I truly felt a sense of appreciation for modern medical treatments. Certainly not for the unloving way in which it was delivered at the hospital, but for the treatment itself and to all the research that must have gone into creating it.

This brings forth a new thought-

What if the same cutting edge lifesaving treatments were delivered with hands of love? With more compassion and tenderness? The kind that Reiki offers.

This sacred balance is an intention for the future.

The Hidden Gems in Unpleasant Experiences

• On the spiritual path, a primary lesson is to take responsibility for everything that appears in our lives. The soul creates its own experiences, both unpleasant and pleasant.

• An unpleasant experience may be karmic in nature. It works to balance out karma between souls and situations. Reiki can speed up karmic cleansing. This helps a soul ascend to a higher level of consciousness with minimal karma to clear.

• Very often, an unpleasant experience is a stepping stone to realize our inherent purpose in divine time.

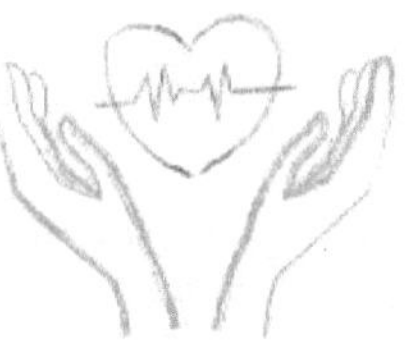

Comfort in Reiki
Suraj

Every little pain and ache,

Does not need medicine to take.

The body can heal a great many ills,

Allow it time, if only one wills.

The last time I took an antibiotic was fifteen years ago for a dental infection. I allow self-limiting illnesses such as a common cold or a flu to run their own course and heal in their own time. Despite being a doctor myself, I rarely take medicines, as most often the body takes care of itself pretty well.

Haripriya kindly offers to give me Reiki every time I am unwell. And I always accept her offer with joy and gratitude.

Every time I receive Reiki, it is a very relaxing experience. I find it so soothing that I drift into peaceful slumber. I love the soft ambience created with warm candles and calming music. I love the gentle presence of Haripriya while she works on 'balancing my chakras' as she calls it. The feeling of being nurtured by a loved one when unwell means the world to me.

Peace and relaxation, gentle presence and healing comfort - this is what I like most about Reiki.

Self-Healing vs External Support

The human body is a natural healer. Most often, it maintains health and balance. It is innately programmed to restore most imbalances independently. For example, most minor injuries heal on their own. Medications used to treat most viral infections are used just to relieve symptoms and not to cure the infection itself. The infection settles in its own time.

Specific treatments are required only when the body is unable to achieve a healing outcome independently. For instance, in the case of major infections, blocked arteries or malignant tumors, it may not be possible to recover without help. And in such situations, it is important to access appropriate healthcare.

From time immemorial, people have turned to different forms of medicine whenever the body needed additional support to heal. The concept of 'Ki' proposes the existence of an energy which gives life to the body and supports its efforts towards healing. And a Reiki session certainly makes one re-vitalized and rejuvenated. Considering these benefits, Reiki is already a part of complimentary care in several hospitals around the world. However, for Reiki to be offered as part of mainstream treatment, more research and concrete evidence is required.

Allowing the body to heal naturally when it can is a sign of strength, while turning to external support when it can't is a sign of wisdom.

Year 2012
Haripriya

As 2012 arrives,

Millions of Angels appear in the skies.

Shining their lights bright and high,

To help every caterpillar emerge a butterfly

As I journeyed on with a more rational perspective in place, I hardly gave Reiki or other metaphysical concepts any thought. However, I was surprised to find myself craving Reiki every once in a while. And I did indulge in Reiki self-healing sessions once every few months, just because I felt like it.

Then came 2011, bringing with it some new challenges. Nothing major but certainly annoying enough to create some imbalances in my life. Unhealed emotions from my past experience of child loss came storming into my awareness. I had been in denial for too long and was being nudged to develop an acceptance of life.

As these emotions gained momentum, I realized I could do little to help myself with the support of my rational mind alone. No logic was of any help to my troubled mind and heart.

The cries of my soul grew louder and louder, until one day in early 2012, I could ignore it no longer. I knew I had to get in touch with my disowned spiritual side again or risk going berserk.

I then began working with a wonderful therapist who helped me heal myself using 'Emotional Freedom Technique' and the 'I AM' meditations. I soon began to feel lighter and brighter, as if I had restored my relationship with a long lost friend.

As I re-established this connection with Spirit, to my utmost astonishment and secret delight, Reiki gradually eased its way back into my life!

One day, I simply knew that Reiki had to be a part of my life again, irrespective of what it could do for me or for others. I took a conscious decision to practice self-healing with no expectations whatsoever. I told myself that the only way to discover what it was would be to explore it with an open mind.

I practiced Reiki every single day in a state of absolute blankness and zero expectation. And at the end of six months, I had evolved from a struggling caterpillar into a soaring butterfly. I had undergone a deep transformation indeed. Nothing tangible, nothing miraculous to flaunt to the outside world. Just a deep inner shift that left me feeling empowered in new ways. I experienced a deeper connection with my body, mind, and Spirit. I discovered a road to not just wellness of the body, but wholeness of the Body, Mind and Spirit.

Sacred 2012

In New Age circles, the year 2012 was considered a harbinger of great change and a significant spiritual milestone for Planet Earth. Consciousness levels would rise, and new ways of life would gradually begin to replace outdated ones.

This time also celebrated the rising of the Divine Feminine energies that honor the rhythm and flow of life. These same energies also inspire one to feel intuitively.

This special year seems to have turned on hidden switches of spiritual wisdom in numerous souls all over the world.

Reiki is undoubtedly one such switch. It serves as a catalyst to activate higher levels of consciousness. A Reiki self-healing balances the flow of the life force, calms the breath and soothes the body and mind. In this meditative state, the doors to our inner world open up, and life is no longer limited to the five senses!

Look back at your own life. Did the year 2012 act as a turning point?

If yes, have you appreciated your heightened pace of spiritual progress since then, and the distance you have come till now?

Have you made note of the soul lessons you have learnt and the victories you have achieved?

Celebrate your journey!

If the answer is no, that's perfectly fine too. All it means is that the energetic shifts relevant for you are happening in the background and you will be aware of them at the appropriate time.

Reiki Takes Centre Stage
Haripriya

The gifts of the feminine begin to shine,

Intuition aplenty and guidance divine.

Life unfolds in perfect time,

Reiki reveals its secrets sublime.

My renewed discovery of Reiki led me into the very depths of my being. My intuition grew stronger and I was flowing in perfect harmony with my life. I allowed whatever served my growth to remain and let go of anything that did not.

I soon felt ready for Reiki Mastership. Receiving the Master attunement took me deeper along the road of spiritual healing.

As I moved ahead with no expectations, Reiki took over the reins and launched me on my life's path.

Life began to unfold spontaneously.

I came in contact with some incredible Spiritual Teachers, who mentored me in the areas of past life healing, inner child healing and chakra healing. During this inner work, I discovered my potential as an energy healer and also my mission here on Earth. There was no looking back after this and I just knew what I had to do to move forward.

Along the way, the beautiful Angel energy also became an integral part of my life and my Reiki practice. Guided by my inner voice, my purpose unfolded on its own.

I soon emerged as a teacher of Reiki and Angel healing. I also blossomed as an author, soon after my intuition led me to the beautiful website Reiki Rays. Writing has always been my passion and I was delighted when this door opened for me.

Balance between Planning and Allowing

One of the principles of the spiritual quest is to allow life to unfold. While the Rational Masculine plans and controls certain aspects of life, the Intuitive Feminine surrenders and allows other aspects to blossom spontaneously. Trying to plan every single detail can be exhausting, as can leaving everything to natural flow. The middle path is where the magic is experienced.

When we allow spontaneity, we invite great beauty, joy and purpose into our lives. The mind can help us plan many things in great detail. When the mind is joined by the heart, it forms a complete team.

With Reiki as a companion on the path, it becomes easier to allow life to just happen. Regular Reiki self-healing helps one travel within oneself. This strengthens the realization that everything will turn out for the highest good and that it is safe to allow the splendors of life to reveal themselves.

Intuition in Everyday Life and Medicine
Suraj

What is this mysterious inner knowing?

That seems to keep life flowing.

When rationality does not find a way,

Intuition steps in with secrets to say.

I used the word 'intuition' very rarely. To me intuition was a combination of subconscious observation, experience and guesswork. However, I found Haripriya using this word on a very frequent basis, especially after 2012. She had discovered a new love and truth in Reiki and was making great personal and professional progress. During this time, she started taking intuitive decisions on an everyday basis. She spoke of knowing about 'what's good' and 'what's not good' under different circumstances. She seemed to be able to tune into the moods and life stories of people without them saying a word. When we had to relocate, she even selected our new home based on the 'vibration' that she felt there.

Another close encounter with her intuition was when she seemed to know that it was time for me to make a career move. She even gave a hint as to which hospital would enhance my professional growth. But at that point, I operated solely from my rational mind and thought her suggestion was unworkable. I also held beliefs about financial remuneration being limited in our city.

But she was confident that the 'Universe' places no limits when one 'vibrates' at the 'frequency' of their desire! This talk of frequency and vibration continued to be unfathomable to me and I did not give it much thought. But surprisingly enough, one fine day, an offer came my way from the very hospital she had mentioned.

All through the process of negotiation and recruitment, she encouraged me to stay on course. She said this hospital carried a nice positive vibration and was a match to my own level of growth. Truly enough, everything worked out well, not just work wise but financially too. And I let go of my previous limiting belief with regard to financial inadequacy.

Though my logical mind tried to rationalize the whole episode, I gave credit to Haripriya's elements of intuition and feminine wisdom that provided a boost to my professional growth.

I am also happy to acknowledge that this book was the outcome of Haripriya's intuition. One day in January 2019, she told me that she had a vision of this book in her morning meditation and asked if I would co-author it. I gave it some thought and decided that sharing our individual perspectives could be beneficial to many readers.

Intuition in Medicine

The word 'intuition' is rarely used in medical terminology. But considering that medicine is both a science and an art, practitioners frequently use their intuition, irrespective of whether they are aware of it or not.

Very often, a doctor knows what to expect from a patient the minute they set foot into the clinic. The subtle signals they give out during their consult and their body language speak volumes to an experienced practitioner. This art of assessment is honed over years of experience. Energy healers would probably call this an 'energy field' emanated by the patient.

Though medical treatments are evidence based, they are often required to be delivered in various permutations and combinations, depending on the case being treated. Many decisions – for example, what is a probable diagnosis (and what could be other possible diagnoses), what treatment to give, what not to give, when to give, when to change it, when to stop, when to operate, when not to operate - are often based on judgement and intuitive decision making.

Many people may not be conscious of the intuition operating in their lives. Nonetheless, it is used by almost everyone in varying degrees.

Unconditional Love: The Merging of the Rational-Masculine and the Intuitive-Feminine
Haripriya and Suraj

Haripriya

As I embraced both my rational and intuitive sides, life moved ahead in leaps and bounds. On the family front, we were blessed with our angelic and adorable baby boy! On the professional front, I began doing work which resonated with my heart and soul. Things couldn't be any better!

But there was always this niggling voice about Suraj in the background.

"Is he still holding on to his closeted reality as the only version of the truth? Will he ever get the essence of the intuitive side?"

There were times when these thoughts troubled my heart. If I spoke to him about it, his views emerged even stronger, which resulted in me feeling angry and let down. Unconsciously, I seemed to be hoping that he would change at least a little bit, after having lived so many years with me.

However, his love for me was always unconditional. He never seemed to expect that I become more rational or change my views. This unconditional love was something I couldn't ignore.

After months of meditating and praying for guidance on why my partner would not modify his views, my intuition said,

"If he can love me as I am, can I not love him as he is?"

This unconditional love sealed our relationship and took it forward. I operated predominantly from intuition and Suraj operated predominantly from rationality, yet both of us embraced the other's perspective whenever required.

We opened up to imbibe whatever is good from the world of medicine and rationality, as well as from the realm of Reiki and intuition.

Some more years rolled past in this manner. In December 2018, I attended an energy healing conference. The speakers spoke about their individual experiences and about how there is a lack of acceptance of their work in mainstream medicine. They also felt that this was mainly because of insufficient research and documentation. Once back home, I shared these viewpoints with Suraj. He immediately offered to share the principles of research and evidence based practice to practitioners of alternative healing who were open to exploring it. He hoped that this would help them conduct research of their own and possibly integrate their services into the mainstream.

This was an aha moment indeed!

Suddenly, it felt like this was the common destination our individual paths had ultimately led up to.

It was the divine purpose of my partner to show me the benefit of rational application in the world, while it was my divine purpose to show him the beauty of intuitive application.

It was the divine purpose of my partner to reach out to others like me, through me, while it was my divine purpose to reach out to others like him, through him.

And now, we see it as our combined purpose to help those on one side appreciate the beauty on the other side, until the lines blur and both sides fuse into one.

The merging of the masculine and the feminine in perfect harmony to birth a whole new world!

For those who would like to tune into their rational side and explore the world of research, Part Two of this book serves as a helpful guide. It includes material shared by Suraj on performing and analyzing scientific research. This knowledge is very close to his heart and soul, as Reiki is to mine. And he shares it with the hope that it will help whoever wishes to empower the domain of alternative therapies.

I trust this book has inspired you to tune into your Rational-Masculine and Intuitive-Feminine sides and to bring out your own unique offering to the world.

Suraj

When Haripriya and I started our journey together, we had no inkling that this is where we would end up ten years down the line!

As always, to me, this is the next logical step that emerged.

Through this piece of work, I hope that practitioners of 'alternative therapies' are able to objectively evaluate research done by others as well as take up research of their own. It is important to understand that outcome based quality evidence can be generated for any kind of healing therapy using the techniques described in Part Two.

I pray that the research efforts of the energy healing community bring great success to them. I also pray that the positive outcomes of research in alternative healing are applied to help millions of people in need.

On a final note, for those who wish to explore their intuitive side and dream big, I encourage you to read Part Three of this book. Haripriya shares some remarkable insights on creating a new system of 'Empowered Medicine'. With both magic and logic as its pillars, the visualization of this new model is sure to spark your imagination. The intention of this visualization is to consciously manifest a magical reality, achieved through the combined power of rationality and intuition.

Oops! My words sound too fairytale-like to my rational ears but as long as it's all for the good, nothing else matters.

Strong rational masculine,

And soft intuitive feminine.

When thee merge in time divine,

Earth and Sky awaken and shine!

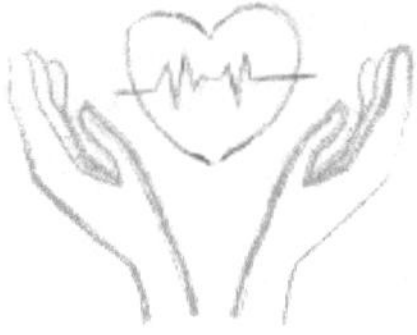

Part 2

Science in Alternative Therapies
An Evidence Based Approach

Suraj Manjunath

Introduction

The intention of this section is to provide insight and inspiration to those practitioners of alternative healing therapies who would like to explore the world of research. The information presented here is to enable practitioners to independently and critically evaluate published research. It may also inspire them to initiate quality research projects of their own, thereby lending greater credibility to their work.

As I understand it, some alternative therapies also act as tools for emotional healing and spiritual growth. When a therapy is used as a personal choice to facilitate emotional health or spiritual growth, it may not need research to validate it. However, research is required when something needs to be executed with exacting standards. It is most certainly required to validate a therapy before it is offered as medical treatment.

The technical knowledge shared in this section is based on the principles of evidence based practice, as applied in medicine today.

Emotional - Spiritual Aspects of Research

The willingness to fail is part of research efforts. More often than not, various trials in science and medicine do not fetch the results hoped for. A large number of drug related trials fail to generate the expected outcome. A drug which showed promising results in the lab may not work when tested on actual patients.

When an experiment fails, it is important not to feel disheartened. In spiritual terms, this would amount to not being attached to the outcome.

Perseverance is key. If an experiment shows that a certain therapy does not offer the kind of benefit that we hoped for, it is not the end of the world. Therefore, it is crucial to persist with ongoing research.

For the greatest benefit to researchers and the world at large, research projects must be undertaken with the following firmly in place-

• The courage to eliminate biases and prejudices, and to explore ideas with an open mind, following the highest standards of scientific inquiry.

• The grace to accept unsuccessful outcomes.

• The spirit to celebrate successful outcomes and to work towards implementing them practically.

• The will to continue research efforts and consistently work towards achieving higher and more improved outcomes.

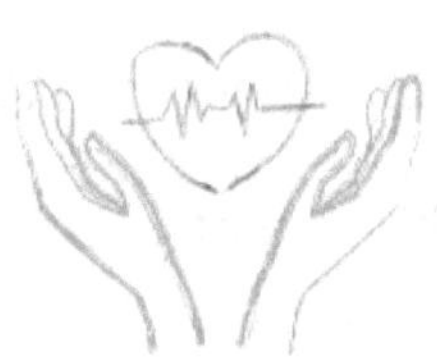

The Core Guiding Principle

A very important guiding principle taught to all medical students is "Primum non nocere", which in Latin means "first, do no harm". It is wiser to do nothing than to do something which would make a sick person worse.

From this tenet of non-maleficence emerges the need for "evidence."

If a doctor/healer offers something to a patient, he should be as certain as possible that it works. The downside of not being certain is that it often creates more harm than good. Even if a particular therapy does not cause direct harm to a patient, it may cause indirect harm by preventing him from taking therapy which would have been more effective.

When in doubt, the principle of *'"Primum non nocere"* acts as a guiding light.

Importance of an Evidence Base

According to the Merriam Webster dictionary, evidence is *'something that furnishes proof'*.

In modern medicine, a fundamental requirement for the regulatory approval of a drug or a therapeutic approach is high quality 'evidence.'

This 'evidence' is the foundation of the modern medical system that is practiced worldwide. It has grown to be an unshakable foundation, that is emerging stronger with time and effort. However, it is interesting to note that things have not always been this way in the history of medicine. This evidence based approach has evolved over a long period of time.

In the early days of medicine, treatments were often based on random ideas and hypothesis. And the results achieved at that time were extremely poor when compared to the outcomes achieved through evidence based research today.

The advances made in medicine till date are the result of the painstaking research efforts of brilliant minds across the globe. These efforts have paid off so well that evidence based medicine brings relief in various forms to millions of people around the globe each day.

As harsh and invasive as modern medicine seems on the surface, the fact remains that the solid evidence base backing this system is working wonders. These include advances in accident and emergency care, cure of many infectious diseases, management of chronic illnesses, maternal and child health care, and complex life-saving surgical procedures.

Compared to conventional medical treatments, alternative therapies undoubtedly offer a gentler approach to healing. They are often based on the principle of 'root cause healing', that is, healing the disease at source and not just its external manifestations. As appealing as the hypothesis sounds, there is a lack of a strong evidence base to demonstrate the efficacy of this approach.

In order for these therapies to be integrated into the mainstream, evidence generated by high quality research is necessary. If a strong evidence base can show the effectiveness of these therapies, it would make sense to employ these gentler approaches to healing wherever applicable.

Therapies based on strong evidence help those who receive it as well as those who practice it, in addition to providing greater authority to the healing community.

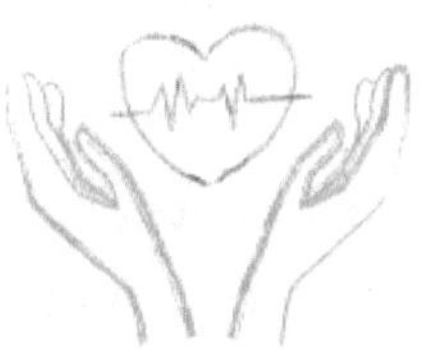

Unlearning and Learning

When learning something new, it often helps to do a bit of unlearning!

While trying to understand 'evidence', it also helps to understand what is not 'evidence.'

1. Hearsay - Casual statements made by people do not constitute evidence. Just because someone says something with conviction, it does not automatically make it valid. There may be partial or complete truth in the story but it does not equate with evidence. For instance, a statement such as "My neighbor's friend tried this particular hair oil which cured his baldness," is not evidence.

2. Posts and forwards on Social media - Where I live, social media is frequently bombarded by messages that offer unverified and unscientific medical information and solutions, thereby misleading many gullible people. Typical messages would go something like this –

> • "The main treatment for cancer is to stop all intake of sugar. Without sugar in your body, the cancer cells die naturally."

> • "The bitterness of Margosa leaves fights the sweetness in sugar and thereby cures diabetes. Chew ten leaves a day and diabetes will be cured in three months."

The people circulating such messages probably have the best of intentions. They may sincerely believe these messages to be true and hope that these posts will help those suffering. Unfortunately, such posts do not constitute evidence. And taking important health related decisions based on social media posts can actually do more damage.

3. Traditional Practices - If a specific treatment has been loosely in practice for a long time and is believed to offer some relief or healing, it does not constitute evidence. For example, the potentially dangerous practice of stopping breast-feeding if a baby develops diarrhoea.

Sometimes however, some practices could be a starting point to look for evidence of its benefit.

4. Fads/ Trends - If some practice suddenly becomes popular among people, it does not constitute evidence. Just because everyone's doing it, does not necessarily mean it works. For example, some kinds of 'detox diets'

5. Individual Opinions - Opinions of individuals based on their personal and subjective experience do not constitute evidence, especially if they are not directly working in the concerned field. Many celebrities may have their own personal opinions regarding what works and what does not. However, their opinion does not constitute evidence, as a result of their celebrity status. For instance, a rocket scientist may have an opinion on the best way to grow vegetables. This does not automatically make it valid, on the grounds that it is the opinion of a leading scientist.

6. Anecdotal - This includes accounts of what happened to someone somewhere at some time. A one-time incident, as miraculous as it may sound, does not constitute evidence. Evidence must be reproducible under all, if not most, circumstances.

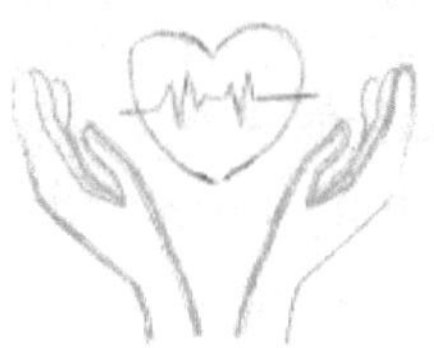

Levels of Evidence

Evidence can be ranked on the basis of the quality and quantity of available and published research studies.

The higher the level of evidence, the more accurate is the proposition.

The factors determining the level of evidence are - demonstrability, reproducibility, high quality of data, and a large quantity of data

Demonstrability

When somebody claims to have achieved something, he should be able to demonstrate it convincingly. For instance, if an energy practitioner says that he can charge a mobile phone through cosmic energy, he should be able to demonstrate it to an impartial audience.

Reproducibility

The outcome claimed by a particular researcher must be reproducible even when done by others. Going back to the example of charging a mobile phone, if one practitioner is able to successfully demonstrate the charging of a mobile phone through cosmic energy, it must also be possible for other energy practitioners to achieve similar outcomes. It may vary in degree but it cannot be that nobody else is able to achieve the same result.

Similarly, a therapy offered to patients in a certain way should produce the same or similar results even when done by other researchers.

When the hypothesis being tested is concrete, such as the charging of a mobile phone, demonstrability and reproducibility can be evaluated easily. However, it may be challenging to demonstrate a difference in outcomes for more subjective conditions, say back pain or migraine. In such cases, more elaborate studies may need to be done.

Quality of data

The lowest quality of evidence is an **individual expert's opinion or a case report.** No clinical recommendation can be made on this basis.

Efforts should be made to progress from this low-level evidence to higher standards like **retrospective case series.**

This should move on to even higher levels like **prospective trials using smaller numbers** (where methodological quality may be poor) to ultimately high quality **prospective randomized controlled trials.**

In clinical research, the 'gold standard' high level evidence is a **multi-centric prospective randomized controlled trial.** It may not always be possible to generate this superior quality of evidence in all circumstances.

It is a good idea to begin research projects on a smaller scale, targeting lower levels of evidence. If a smaller study generates a successful outcome, the hypothesis can then be more rigorously tested through prospective analysis or randomized controlled trials.

To quote an example from medical history - an infection of the gallbladder (cholecystitis) is a serious illness which has claimed many lives in the past. The main treatment is surgical removal(cholecystectomy) which was done by open conventional surgery for more than a hundred years since 1882. In the mid-1980s, a few surgeons in Europe individually performed keyhole (laparoscopic) cholecystectomies on a few patients. Initially, their reports were received with skepticism. Gradually, more evidence emerged in the form of case series (low level evidence), followed by case control studies (higher level evidence) and followed even later by randomized controlled studies which established the superiority of laparoscopic cholecystectomy. Today, this technique has replaced open cholecystectomy as the gold standard for removal of gall bladder.

Quantity of Data

The more the number of trials that are conducted for a certain therapy, the more reliable the data. If more groups of researchers show similar results for a therapy, it is much more likely that the particular therapy will benefit the majority of patients when applied.

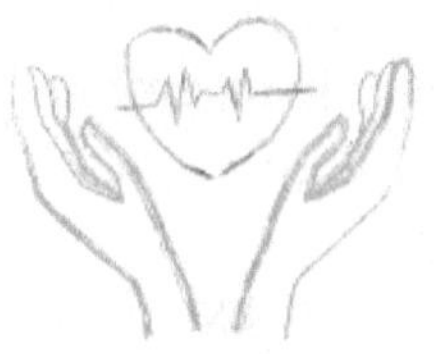

Process of Generating Evidence

We will now look into the various steps that go into the process of gathering data and generating evidence.

Choosing a research topic

A study should ideally be done on an issue which is common enough, and is relevant to society. Once such a topic is identified, all existing information about it, including previously conducted research should be meticulously studied. A new study should be designed on this basis.

Formulating a Research question

A good way to begin a study is by posing a question. The end result of the study would be the answer to this question. The question should be as specific and measurable as possible.

Let us assume the topic to be studied is essential hypertension (the common variety of elevated blood pressure) – a widespread and an important healthcare issue. And let us assume that the intervention we want to study is the effect of Reiki healing on reducing blood pressure in hypertensives. We can design a study involving two groups- one group receives Reiki healing and the other receives therapy which resembles Reiki healing but is not (placebo). The receiver will not know which one he has received.

A research question such as *"Does Reiki help with healing hypertension?"* is a poorly designed question.

A better question would be *"Do Reiki sessions given thrice a week for an hour each time, taken over three months, reduce the blood pressure readings **significantly** as compared to placebo, in a population of patients with essential hypertension?"*

The frequency and duration of the sessions themselves should be decided by Reiki experts on the basis of previous experience and already published smaller series which have discussed these technicalities.

Please note that the word 'significant' has a specific meaning in the context of research – it does not denote magnitude or importance. The term 'significant' in research means that the difference in outcome between study groups is more than what can be explained by chance. We'll come to that again later.

In the second research question asked above, the possible answers are either 'yes' or 'no'. Sometimes, even if the answer to a particular study question is 'no', a detailed analysis of the study could lead to other potential questions that merit further research.

For example, assuming the answer to the Reiki in hypertension question is 'no', deeper analysis may reveal that elderly women alone appeared to benefit. So, it may be worth further studying the effect of Reiki in hypertension in that particular subset of patients, by designing a new study.

Randomization

As discussed earlier, the highest levels of evidence are generated from randomized controlled trials. Here there are two or more groups of participants.

Participants are randomly assigned to study groups using various techniques - essentially flipping a coin for each participant to determine which group he goes to. This ensures that every group has a wide variety of people and helps in the elimination of bias while formulating groups.

A group receives either no therapy or different doses/frequency of therapy.

Power of a Study

It is important that a research study is designed with enough power, meaning, it includes a substantial number of participants. This will enable the research question to be answered with greater certainty.

If a throw of dice numbered one to six, lands on the number six twice in a row, it is most likely just due to chance. If it lands on six, ten consecutive times, it is more likely that the dice is modified in some way. It could still be due to chance, but that is less likely. If the same dice lands on six, a hundred times consecutively, then it is almost certain that it is not due to chance.

In the same way, if a therapy is offered to very few people, it may be difficult to say whether any improvement is due to the therapy itself or the result of chance or something else.

The number of study subjects needed for a reasonably powered study depends on what is being studied and how much variation is expected in outcomes. A good statistician is needed to calculate this.

Reports of single cases, or small series of cases are therefore low level evidence, although it could serve as a starting point to conduct better research.

Prospective versus Retrospective Studies

Retrospective analysis is fraught with biases. Here the study is not based on pre-defined parameters.

For example, if a study retrospectively analyses patients with advanced pancreatic cancer who received a particular type of chemotherapy, it may show that they survived longer than those who didn't receive it. However, it could be possible that the patients who received chemotherapy and could tolerate it, were healthier and fitter and were likely to live longer anyway.

A *prospective study* reduces biases. In this, we define the parameters of the study beforehand – the number of subjects to be recruited (power of the study), what intervention is going to be applied, how much, how frequently, and for how long. Also, the outcomes that are going to be studied are defined beforehand, and not at the end of the study.

Association and Causation

Let us understand this concept with a hypothetical example. A black colored car is more likely to be involved in an accident because of reduced visibility against a dark road surface and lower visibility at night. So, the color black is associated with increased risk of accidents and is also a cause.

A red car may also be more prone to an accident. But it could be because a person buying a red car is more likely to be younger and a risk taker. In this case, the color red is associated with increased risk of accidents but is not a cause. In fact, a red car may be better visible than duller colors and in itself actually reduce the risk of accidents.

Applying this concept to healing, a person who is more open to undergo a specific form of energy therapy, may also be more inclined to presume that there has been a positive change. Therefore, it is important to evaluate whether the improvement is an association or a causation. The next section shows us how to overcome this bias.

Blinding of a Study

Blinding is the process of withholding information that may prejudice study participants or data collectors in some way. For example, if a group of people **know they are** receiving a particular energy therapy for gastro-esophageal reflux (heartburn), they may be more likely to feel better compared to another group who **know they are not** receiving it. Also, if the person collecting data already knows that a particular subject has received the actual therapy, he may be biased to record an improvement even if there is none.

A trial is called 'single blind' when just one group is blinded, normally the participants of the study.

A trial is called 'double blind' when both the participants and those who collect the data are blinded. In a double-blind trial studying the 'Reiki in Hypertension' hypothesis described above, no individual participant must know what they received. In addition, the people questioning the participants after Reiki healing/placebo, should be unaware of who received what.

After data collection is complete, the trial is unblinded- that is, the evaluators now know which participant received what and who showed improvement. The data is then analyzed to look for any statistically significant difference in outcome between the two groups.

Statistical Tests of Significance

These are mathematical tools that validate the outcomes of a study and reduce the possibility of a chance outcome. Good studies involve a statistician right from the time of study design until analysis and conclusion. For those good at math, there are also many online tools available to help with this.

Fishing expedition

If I throw a fishing line and come up with a random fish, I can always claim that was the exact fish I was looking for!

When doing a study, the outcome to be measured should be defined beforehand. Inevitably, when large amounts of data are analyzed, there is bound to be some difference or the other among study groups, which may be irrelevant to the actual outcome being studied. Unless that difference was meant to be looked for beforehand, it is of no consequence.

Let's say a trial is done to see if a particular therapy helps with weight loss. Towards the end of the study, it is found that there is no difference as far as weight loss is concerned. On detailed evaluation done in hindsight, someone notices that statistically significant number of participants in one group took a vacation the month following the therapy. It definitely cannot be concluded that therapy helped them go on a vacation! If at all somebody feels that this is a possibility, a new study should be designed to see if this therapy helps people go on vacation.

Final Analysis of a Study

Once data evaluation is complete, the outcomes have to be analyzed in context. The question that we posed initially as an example was-

"Do Reiki sessions given thrice a week for an hour each time, taken over three months, reduce the blood pressure readings significantly as compared to placebo, in a population of patients with essential hypertension?"

If the answer to this is 'yes' based on a well conducted prospective randomized double blind controlled trial of enough power, then it means we have enough evidence to say,

"Reiki does help with healing hypertension."

And the more the number of such trials showing similar results, the better the evidence.

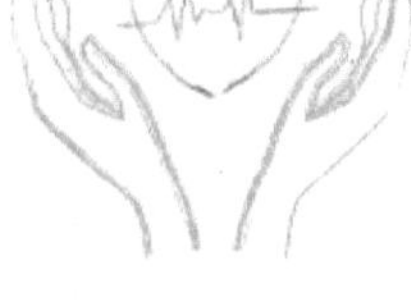

Conclusion

Conducting research as well as critically evaluating others' research can be a very rewarding experience. Apart from stimulating the mind, it also helps in the practical application of therapies and services. Research helps uncover the numerous mysteries of the Universe. It guides us towards new potential and possibilities, thereby helping current and future generations.

I hope you enjoyed this brief exploration of the world of research. This is just the starting point. I trust this piece of work has enriched your knowledge. I am optimistic that your enhanced understanding of this subject will inspire your own research efforts.

Wishing you great success!

Part 3

Empowered Medicine
A Spiritual Approach

Haripriya Suraj

Introduction

This section is for the day dreamers and the master creators! It is about dreaming a new system of healing into being, through focused intention, guided action and divine support. Today this system may exist primarily in the imagination. But the imagination can be a powerful starting point for any new creation.

Features of the New System

• It incorporates the best of Spirit and Science, the best of intuitive wisdom and evidence based practice

• It is a seamless interconnection of different healing services, all working with the common intention of offering healing in loving and empowered ways. Wellness therapies, energy health services, preventive healthcare, medical, surgical and emergency care are all offered under the same roof.

• It allows doctors and energy healers to work hand in hand, each taking their rightful place and contributing their unique strengths to the process of healing.

The good news is that many healthcare centers around the globe are already open to newer possibilities. They offer therapies which are currently termed 'non-conventional' as complimentary care services. This is a great starting point. However, there is still work to do.

Pre-requisites for the New System

• The responsibility of creating this new system does not depend on the healthcare sector alone. It is dependent on the whole population.

• Levels of consciousness in the human race must rise to a higher threshold, which means both the people offering healing as well as those receiving it must operate from empowerment and not in victim consciousness.

• Those in the giver's position must work because it resonates true to them and brings joy to their soul. They must not work just because someone told them to do so.

• Those in the receiver's position must feel empowered enough to receive healing in complete awareness. They must be willing to take responsibility and feel no need to blame doctors, healers or external circumstances for their health.

• People must connect with their bodies and be inspired to work to maintain balance in all areas of their lives. However, they must also be willing to receive the support of healthcare when required.

• Modern medicine becomes more humane. Advanced research helps develop technology that makes medical interventions more pleasant.

• Alternative therapies cultivate a concrete evidence base. They are no longer viewed as 'complimentary' but as an essential component to the overall process of healing.

Since many factors need to come together for this creation, it may not work for everyone in the current time period. But let us intend that it starts off now for everybody that feels the calling - for those doctors, healers, healthcare administrators and regulatory authorities that feel ready to create such a model and for the people who feel ready to receive from it.

One step at a time is all that is needed……

And the future will automatically take care of itself.

Let us intend that this model becomes reality for Planet Earth. Let us intend that the levels of consciousness rise so high that every creation reflects this level!

The pillars of this new system of empowered medicine are-

Comprehensive Healing Centre

Nurturing Doctor/Healer

Empowered Patient

Let us explore each of these pillars some more.

Comprehensive Healing Center

The hospital of the new system will be a comprehensive healing center with medical personnel and energy practitioners, all operating in a high vibrational environment.

A hospital is a space associated with healing. Logically speaking, going to a hospital must bring a sense of relief to ailing patients. However, many people find the very thought of visiting a hospital unpleasant. Some go to great lengths to avoid going as it induces a sense of fear in them.

On the contrary, visiting an energy healing center isn't a scary experience for most people. It usually creates feelings of peace, safety and hope in them.

What if the same safe and nurturing environment of energy healing centers is also created in hospitals?

When a patient walks into a comprehensive healing center, he enters a serene space with positive energy flowing through it. Imagine a space adorned with warm scented candles, fresh flowers, healing crystals and calming music filling the air! Such a center also has outdoor spaces with plenty of greenery and water bodies adding to its beauty.

The workforce at such a center radiate compassion. They are kind yet know how to be firm when required. They are present in this space because they love to do this work. They are tuned in to their source of inner strength. The environment is a beautiful symphony of calmness, love, strength, and healing.

Irrespective of whether someone walks in to this center for a yoga class, a Reiki session or a surgical procedure, they are met by the same positive vibration everywhere. Every space in this center offers the same feelings of safety and comfort.

The clinics and procedure rooms are gentle and nurturing spaces that are also equipped with the necessary medical technology. Despite the presence of complex medical equipment, patients feel at ease because the levels of consciousness in the space are high.

The birthing rooms are special and comforting spaces to give birth. They are bright, cheery and warm. The expectant mother is treated as a Goddess and is nurtured with love. Every baby that is born is received by gentle and welcoming hands.

Energy therapies supported by a strong evidence base are integrated into the system wherever appropriate. For example, a pregnant woman may also be offered Yoga classes as part of pre-natal care. A patient could participate in a meditation session before a surgical procedure and perhaps receive Reiki to assist with post-operative recovery.

Patients receive the cream of both worlds, as best suited for a given condition. Holistic healing is adopted as a practice across all specialties of healing. Patients are encouraged to follow the body's natural healing rhythms whenever possible. Medicines and medical treatments are offered when the body needs support to heal. This principle is accepted and followed with ease.

This high vibrational comprehensive healing center is a 'Temple of Healing'. Everyone who visits it leaves healed in body, mind and Spirit.

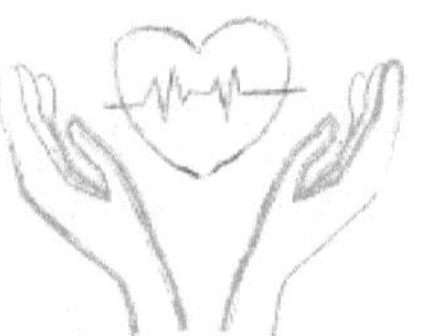

Nurturing Doctor/Healer

In the new system, medicine or healing is not just another profession that people choose. It is a whole new way of life. This work is part of their life purpose and an act of service to humanity.

The following act as guiding principles for the doctors and healers of the new system-

Nurturing with Boundaries

Caregivers master the art of empathetic bonding with souls in pain. At the same time, they are detached enough not to get emotionally involved themselves. They know how to connect so that patients feel safe and comfortable. They nurture patients with compassion because it is the right thing to do, yet honor every patient as a self-empowered being.

Self-Care

Medicine and healing are professions that involve a lot of giving. Too much of giving can be exhausting and can lead to burnout. Therefore, self-care is essential for caregivers as well. Self-care involves getting adequate rest, recreation and replenishment.

Caregivers draw clear energetic boundaries for themselves. They give their best to others on the job but also make it a point to replenish themselves on a regular basis. As self-care becomes a priority, they experience more contentment in their work.

Harmony at Work

Caregivers from different branches of healing work hand in hand. There are no ego clashes or feelings of one discipline being superior to another. Everybody comes together to formulate the best combination of therapies in a given context for a particular patient.

Spiritual Insight

Doctors and healers are well informed about the multi-dimensional nature of health (physical, mental, emotional, social and spiritual as defined by the World Health Organization). The essence of different healing modalities is applied for comprehensive healing of the patient.

Empowered Patient

In the new system, a patient is not just a victim who is afflicted by an illness. He is someone who, despite the illness, is in tune with his body, mind and Spirit. He considers illness an opportunity for growth and views himself as an empowered patient.

The following are the qualities of the 'Empowered Patient'-

Strength and Acceptance

An empowered patient taps into his inner reservoir of spiritual strength to accept things as they are, and he works towards healing himself in appropriate ways.

Illness often creates emotional reactions of denial, anger, bargaining, depression and acceptance (the Kubler-Ross Model). The patient is spiritually conscious and works through these stages, until he is able to reach the state of acceptance and empowerment.

Ability to trust and receive

An empowered patient is able to trust those who treat him and does not feel the need to micromanage the process of healing. He is well informed about the healing being offered to him and wise enough to allow the experts to do their work.

He allows himself the time and space to receive all the healing that he needs. He is not in a hurry to complete the process and rush back into his daily routine. He views this illness as an opportunity for healing, reflection and spiritual growth. He allows himself to be nurtured and cared for by others and emerges stronger through all of it.

He is also pragmatic enough to understand that things may not always turn out the way he expects and feels no need to blame others when a positive healing outcome is not achieved. He is empowered by spiritual wisdom to know that healing is not always about curing. He is able to surrender to the journey even in the face of uncertainty.

Gratitude

An empowered patient adopts an attitude of gratitude. He acknowledges the pain of the illness but also feels grateful for everything else that is working well for him. This could include being grateful for other positive aspects of his health, social support and access to good healthcare.

On a spiritual level, he feels grateful to his body for showing him what needs to be worked on and healed.

This attitude of gratitude shifts the energy in a positive direction and allows effective healing to take place.

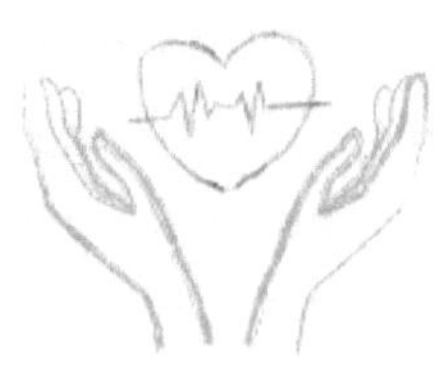

Conclusion

I trust you enjoyed this brief tour into the realm of Empowered Medicine!

"Alone we can do so little; together we can do so much."- Helen Keller.

Let us join hands to make this vision come true. Let us also ask for divine support to birth this new system of Empowered Medicine into being.

With immense love, hope and gratitude in my heart, I conclude this section with a short prayer.

Divine love and light, we call upon thee!

To build a New Earth,

And a New System of Healing to be.

Divine love and light, we call upon thee!

To illuminate the middle path,

In all its wondrous glory.

High vibe and comprehensive healing,

Nurturing giver and empowered receiver.

To lend thy support to this new creation

Oh great Divinity, we humbly call upon thee!

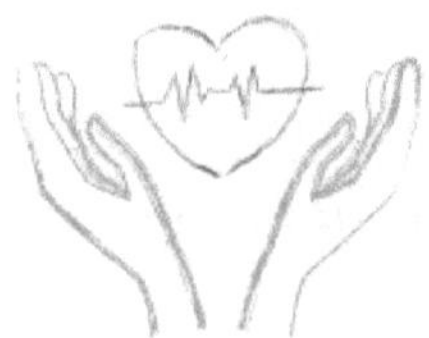

About the Authors

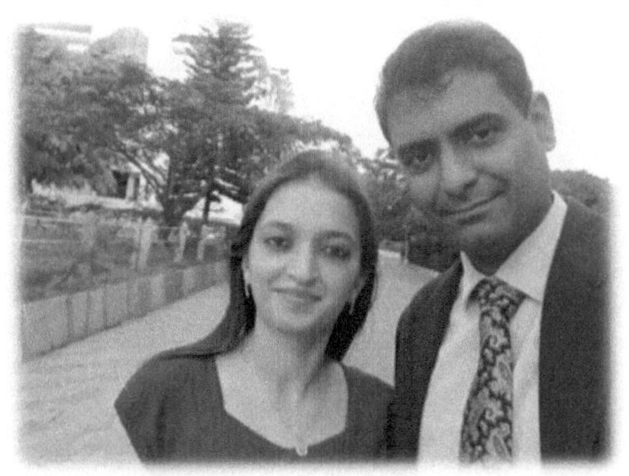

Haripriya & Suraj

Haripriya Suraj *is a Reiki master and an Angel healer. Her first encounter with Reiki happened in her childhood. This set the stage for her life that is largely inspired by Reiki and intuitive wisdom. She adopts a magical approach to life and delights in exploring subtle mysteries of the Universe. Along with practicing Reiki, she also imbibed elements of rationality and scientific thinking. She is now happy to embrace the best of both worlds and finds immense joy in walking the middle path.*

Suraj Manjunath *is a practicing cancer surgeon and a professor of surgical oncology. Rational and scientific in his outlook, he takes the logical route to excellence. Research and evidence based practice are his passions. He advocates the rigorous testing of every hypothesis before presenting it as fact to* *the world. His journey also exposed him to the concepts of energy and intuition and inspired him to help bridge the worlds of Spirit and Science.*

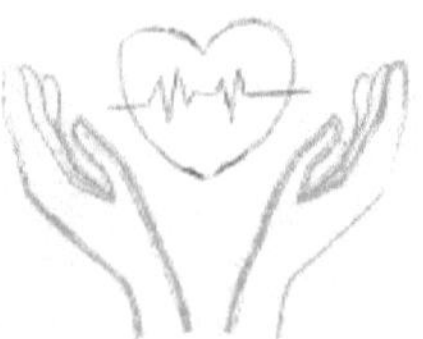

www.ingramcontent.com/pod-product-compliance
Lightning Source LLC
Chambersburg PA
CBHW031143250726
48655CB00002B/808